# The Easiest Diet in the World...
# AND IT WORKS!

## 2ND EDITION

## RICH STEVENS

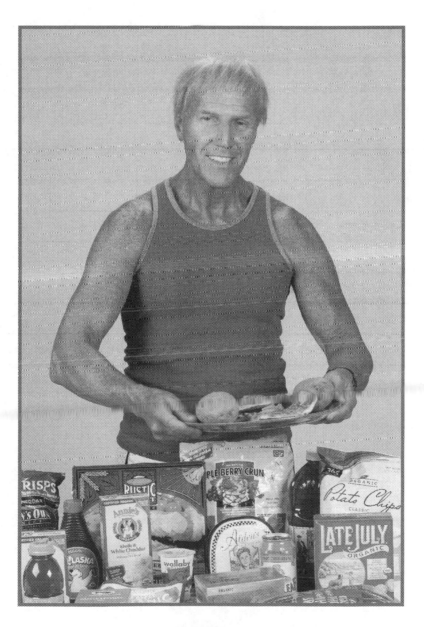

authorHOUSE®

*AuthorHouse™*
*1663 Liberty Drive*
*Bloomington, IN 47403*
*www.authorhouse.com*
*Phone: 1-800-839-8640*

*First published by AuthorHouse 9/7/2011*

*ISBN: 978-1-4520-8631-6 (e)*
*ISBN: 978-1-4520-8630-9 (sc)*

*Library of Congress Control Number: 2010914907*

*Printed in the United States of America*

*This book is printed on acid-free paper.*

*Because of the dynamic nature of the Internet, any Web addresses or links contained in this book may have changed since publication and may no longer be valid. The views expressed in this work are solely those of the author and do not necessarily reflect the views of the publisher, and the publisher hereby disclaims any responsibility for them.*

# Dedication

To all my friends. I hope you read and follow my suggestions here and stay as my happier and healthier friends for a good many more years!

# Acknowledgements

The author wishes to thank his many friends who have given him the impetus to actually publish this book. I wish to thank Paul Gustafson, Bill Lyons, Robert Parker, Bob Mayerhofer, Floyd Holt, and Dee Winter for their advice and help during the nine months that he wrote this book and visited the country getting input.

Also special thanks go out to Robert Bragg for giving the author the final push. As Bob said in his own words "Make this your new love and life. Show everyone your passion for this and make it your impact on society. Go out and tell your amazing story to people. In that way they will get healthier and happier and you'll have fun and be excited too in the process." Without this final push this book would never have been accomplished!

Writing this book was an adventure for me as I have never written a book before and never dreamed I would undertake such a task. But it was as easy as staying on the diet is and as easy as wanting to maintain this lifestyle is! I know that I was inspired and led to do all of this through God's help and guidance! Thank you!!

All photos in this book were not enhanced in any manner and were photographed in September of 2010, by Bela Dornon Studio, located in eastern San Diego. Bela Dornon Studio has been finding a beautiful photo in every face for ten years. www.sdfaceplace.com.

# About The Author

Rich Stevens currently resides in San Diego, California where since 2004 he has served as an adjunct professor of mathematics at Cuyamaca College in El Cajon California.

Rich is a graduate of The State University of New York at Albany where he earned his BA and MA degrees in Math Education. Previous to his move to San Diego in 2001 he taught high school mathematics for his entire teaching career at Franklin Delano Roosevelt High School in Hyde Park New York.

In New York State, Rich also worked as a radio disc jockey weekends on numerous Hudson Valley radio stations playing top 40, oldies, and even doing a talk show. He coached cross country and track at both FDRHS for four years and at Marist College in Poughkeepsie, New York for twelve years. He also served as weight training advisor at FDRHS for ten years. His most prestigious job was as the public address announcer of the New Jersey Nets professional basketball team for seven years in the New Jersey Meadowlands Arena. He has been an avid long distance runner besides coaching distance running at both the high school and collegiate levels. He also organized and directed the Marist College Distance Running Camp with Marty Liquori for eight years.

Rich has been a proponent of physical fitness and has used many techniques in body development, nutrition, health, and fitness. He has experimented with many of the standard techniques developed by others in body weight reduction and healthier lifestyles, all to varying degrees of success.

Moreover, in the last year, due to this new successful lifestyle change, Rich was even asked to model for two national studios. In both cases, he was the oldest person ever asked to model by these two professional photographers! Rich is even featured as "Mr. July" in the 2010 calendar for classicmanphoto.com.

# Contents

# Foreword

Congratulations on your making the decision to buy this book. That is assuming you have actually paid for it and not just stolen it (in which case at least I thank you for thinking it was worthy of that illegal activity!)

The next thing though is to read the entire book and then to activate your own new lifestyle as outlined in this book. I never thought I would write a book ever in my lifetime. And as you will read in this book, I only did so when strongly urged by my friends. Finally one friend practically forced me to write it!

According to the United States Centers for Disease Control and Prevention "American society has become 'obesogenic,' characterized by environments that promote increased food intake, non-healthful foods, and physical inactivity. Policy and environmental change initiatives that make healthy choices in nutrition and physical activity available, affordable, and easy will likely prove most effective in combating obesity." This book is just one step toward that goal!

The obesity trend is getting even alarmingly worse in this country! During the past 20 years there has been a dramatic increase in obesity in the United States. In 2009, only Colorado and the District of Columbia had a prevalence of obesity less than 20%. Thirty-three states had a prevalence equal to or greater than 25%; nine of these states (Alabama, Arkansas, Kentucky, Louisiana, Mississippi, Missouri, Oklahoma, Tennessee, and West Virginia) had a prevalence of obesity equal to or greater than 30%.

I was someone who was not obese or even fat. But I wanted to lose 5-15 pounds and my bulging "love-handles" waistline. What the methods in this book did are beyond my wildest dreams! I never expected what was to take place in the next 4-6 months of time! That is why I do not even have any "before" pictures of myself. The lifestyle change outlined here is explained in details so you will understand the reasons why it works and how it will work for you. It dramatically changed my weight, looks, and health. I receive positive comments and complements every day from both acquaintances and strangers. In the book I even tell about some of these very bold complements I have received from complete strangers.

It is just as the title of the book says. It <u>IS</u> the <u>Easiest</u> Diet in the World ...and It <u>Does</u> Work. And you can eat anything you want! Therefore because of all the positive and great things that will happen to you, and because you do not have to give up eating things you love, you will never EVER want to stop this lifestyle change! You will never go back to your old self. My weight the last three years now is always within three pounds of what I reduced to. This is what I call my "ideal weight". In other diet plans, you eventually lose motivation in the diet, go back to your old eating habits gradually, and gain back those pounds.

In the book I explain why the method works, how you will accomplish it, where to buy foods, what to do when you are traveling and away from home for a while, what restaurants fit in with the lifestyle and what to eat there, and how to save money in your food purchases. I also tell you how to complement the diet part of the lifestyle change with other ideas that will even more dramatically improve the "new you" and make you even more amazing in your new look. I know they always say people don't want to make changes or even change at all. But these are changes you will gladly want to make and then keep forever!

You, the proud owner of this book, also have the contents of the inside pocket "yellow jacket". This jacket contains one page of the important points of the book, as well as logs and charts you can use. I recommend using these logs and charts to help you stay on course and also to help motivate you along the program's path. I recommend reading the entire book first. I do not recommend that you just read those important tips and then decide to start right in with the program. The book will explain why the lifestyle will work and as you read it, you can underline or highlight what is important to you too. But the Important Points Pocket Jacket Page will be useful to keep those strongest points always in mind. The book is a good and quick read. You will understand what the lifestyle change did to me and why it works. You will realize why it will work for you too whether you are just slightly overweight as I was, or even if you are fat or obese. And you will stay with the program the rest of your life. For it is....
The Easiest Diet In The World And It Works!

<u>Answer to the Question under the back cover photo:</u>

When this untouched photo was taken by Bela Dornon Studio in September of 2010, I was 64 years old. How close did you come with your guess? When people meet me, most guess

45-50 years of age, making me LOOK 15-20 years younger than my actual age number. Contained in these pages is more about this "possibility" of yet another benefit of following these guidelines mentioned in this book and what they can do for your face and body as well.

So can following these guidelines make you LOOK younger? Perhaps so! I GUARANTEE that you will FEEL younger and your body LOOKS younger and perhaps even your FACE appears younger if you follow and stay with these guidelines.

# CHAPTER 1

## Oh No! Another Diet Book! Why THIS One is Different!

I know what you are thinking already! Oh no! It's another one of those diet books! Like we really need another one! There must be hundreds of them -produced every week even! Even I was hesitant to write this book! Why wouldn't I be! I had never even written a book before and had no idea how to go about it. But I was so enthused about the amazing things that had happened to me since I started out on my new lifestyle in 2007 and it had changed me in so many unbelievable ways, that I HAD to write a book! I would say to my friends "I should write a book!" And they would mildly say "Yes you should!"

But then one close friend of mine when I said "I should write a book about my change" grabbed my shirt and pulled me toward him and looked at me in the eyes and said "YES! You SHOULD write a book!' And I looked back at him and for three or four seconds we just starred in silence and then I thought for a moment and realized that I should. And here it is now!

So what makes this book and this "diet" different from all the rest of those diet books? Well two things! First, It is sooooo simple! Unlike all the others, I eat anything that I want.... anything! Pasta, potatoes, desserts, ice cream (boy do I love ice cream!), candies, cookies, cakes, brownies, and yes the usual veggies and fruits too. Anything! And second - it works! I KNOW it works beyond my wildest dreams!

In the next chapter I will outline my past experiences with trying to lose weight and diets and dietary supplements. I must admit, only once in my lifetime was I really overweight. The other times I was just someone who wanted to lose 5-15 pounds and lose those love handles. But this diet, or lifestyle as I should really call it, will work for anyone: from those of you who are just slightly overweight and want to lose a few pounds (5-15 pounds) or those who are really overweight and even those who are "obese". And I can safely and modestly say: I GUARANTEE IT!!

So why is it that the rest of those diets DON'T work? Well many work for a while, but then you shift back to your old self and regain back all those pounds you lost through eating a special diet of just certain kinds of things. And many times they are things you don't even want to eat, like grapefruit or eggs or whatever the fad is then. Many of those famous diets were so highly praised when they first came out. But later they were found to be deficient in many nutrients or the logic behind them was proven to be deficient. So you are back where you started and have spent a lot of money on special items and have even lost time. You also have hindered your health with yo-yo poundage going up and down and up and down!

But with this diet you eat whatever you want and you will never ever even want to stray away from it! You will lose the weight amazingly and stay with the same ideal weight the rest of your life! It is so easy and you won't even consider it to be a diet. Again I would call it a "lifestyle" change!

So why did I decide to write this book? Well it will definitely benefit you and I will take pleasure in hearing from you about all the changes -all good I am sure- that have happened to you since you made the change. I will feel fulfilled with just that. But yes, I suppose I will make some money from the books sold too! Also by your going to this lifestyle it will help me and others who are already doing it. It will also bring down the price of the items mentioned here and make those items more abundantly available in more stores. So those are my own honest but selfish reasons too. By your going to this lifestyle change, it will help me and others out too!

Now about my amazement with what has happened to me since making this change back in 2007. I never thought all of this would happen to me. I was so surprised and never expected all of this to happen! That is why I do not even have any "before" pictures to include here! This new lifestyle has put me in the best shape of my life, the best body of my life, and the best health of my life without question! Let me tell you just a few of the stories I have heard from others (who were complete strangers to me) when they saw me and talked with me.

I went on a vacation to Orlando Florida back in 2009 and arrived at the Orlando International Airport around midnight. I had to take a small shuttle bus from the rental car agency to the rental car office. I was the only passenger on this bus, so I sat near the front in the front seat near the bus operator, who was a man in his forties. I asked him just a few procedural questions like "Will there be much of a line at the office" etc. After talking with him for less than a minute, he turned around and looked at me and asked "How old are you?" Now you must be thinking that is quite a bold thing to ask a stranger and also someone who is a client of your firm. But I am now used to such a question from complete strangers. I was going to answer him, but just smiled and was amused at the frequency that I hear this question, so I asked him "Why do you ask that"? He said "Because you are in great shape and I guess probably older than you look". I told him that I was 62 at the time and he said "Man, you have the body of a 20-year old!" Now I do not know how he could really say that. I mean I wasn't naked! I was wearing a form-fitting shirt (not a tank top) and some loose shorts. But I was wearing clothes!! I told him about my lifestyle change for the next 5 minutes or however long it took us to get to the rental car office. He said he would like to do the same thing as he had some health issues and also was overweight. I hope he did the change and perhaps is even reading this now and saying "Hey! He is talking about me! I remember that guy!"

Another time I was walking on the college campus where I teach math and I didn't notice that there was a bench to my right about 20-30 yards and a college-aged guy sitting on it. The next thing I heard was a voice yelling out to me "Hey how old are you"? Again how strange for a student (who I never had in class and still haven't) to yell out and ask THAT as the very first thing blurted out from his mouth. I went over to him and asked "Why do you ask that"? And he said "Cuz you are in good shape"! Again I was not wearing anything that would really show off my body-some loose fitting warm-up pants and a form-fitting shirt I think. I told him I was 61 at the time. He said "Man, you are in VERY good shape then"! I should have told him that he should take my course because he will definitely get an A with those kinds of remarks made to me!

A third and final story occurred September 2009 when I was going to a festival in San Francisco, California. When I was walking around through the crowds of thousands of people, a man in his forties called me over and asked if I had taught high school math in Hyde Park, New York. Of course I had! So I knew he must have been a former student of mine. He was a former student and he remembered me. We hadn't seen each other in over 25 years! And he also did not know I would be there and we never communicated in any form in all those years. After we chatted for about 10 minutes I walked away. Then I thought to myself "Wait a minute! How did he know it was me? That was over 25 years ago and he didn't even know I would be here in San Francisco, let alone at this festival with thousands of people here!" So I went back over to where he had walked and asked him. "Hey how did you recognize me in this crowd of people?" He said "You haven't changed. You look the same!" Wow! What a complement at age 63 and after all those 25+ years! Staying fit and trim does wonders! Maybe even this new lifestyle has made my face look better too-is that possible? More on that later on!

Now I have gotten complements on my body and especially my chest all my life since I started doing weight training when I was in my twenties. But never ever have I received any complements or raves about my stomach. But since I am in the bragging mood right now and talking about complements here, I was thoroughly amazed during 2009 when I actually even received two complements about my stomach. One was in the form of an email I received from a guy who asked if I was at a certain place the day before. When I said yes and asked why, he said "Cuz you have a banging stomach"! Now I was not sure what a "banging" stomach actually meant, but I have since learned that it is a complement! And also while doing one of my walks in San Diego some other guy complemented me and said I looked good and said I had a good stomach! So the new lifestyle has even gotten me complements on what had always been my weakest area...my stomach!

Also as I will outline in this book, I do a very pleasant and fun-filled hour walk every day around my San Diego area. Since "Sun" Diego, as I call it, is very comfortable weather year-round, I often do it shirtless. I get many cars honking their horns (not because they almost hit me) and people yelling (complementary things) out their windows at me. One time a guy, who was one of three friends coming out of a restaurant, even bowed down on the sidewalk as I was walking by!

All these things have happened and I never thought in my wildest dreams I would ever evolve into this apparently good-looking guy with a "hot" body! And especially so when I was in my 60s! I also have been asked by 2 websites now to model for them at age 63 and 64 and I am the oldest model ever used by both of these professional photographers!

So for all the above amazing stories and also for the dramatic changes in my statistics and health, I would never ever consider going back or away from my lifestyle change.

# CHAPTER 2

## My Past Experiences in Diets/Health...and My Body!

I think it is important to outline for you now what "type" of body I have had all my life and my past experience with trying to lose weight and diets. As a kid under 10 years of age, my mother was always worried about me being sickly and I was a "skinny" (or to be "kind") "thin" guy. Then as a teenager I was what I would call a young guy of "average" body frame and weight. But then it happened.

I went to the State University of New York at Albany as an aspiring (and sometimes perspiring) prospective math teacher. And boy did my body change- for the worse! At SUNYA, as it was called then, you got 3 all-you-can-eat buffets for breakfast, lunch, and supper and did I get my money's worth! Eat I did! And besides that, every night I would also get a tuna fish submarine sandwich from Walt's Submarines (later called Big Dom's) and/or half a pizza from Antonio's Pizza. That was way too much (and also weigh too much) meals!!

My weight "blossomed" to over 200 pounds on a guy who is six feet tall. I was definitely overweight and perhaps you could even say FAT!!! And I did no cardio exercise or exercise of any kind! No weight-lifting!

After graduating at SUNYA I decided to lose some weight (and even got contact lenses and did away with my black-rimmed eyeglasses). I ran every day that summer of 1968 on the SUNYA all-weather track. Eventually I did an hour run every day. That was a good thing because when I started teaching at Franklin Delano Roosevelt High School in Hyde Park,

New York I was asked to be the cross country coach of all things! Imagine had I been the fat guy I was 3 months earlier telling all those teenage boys to run long distance!

So actually, there was a lifestyle change at age 22 for me. No more eyeglasses and no more fatness. Now instead I was looking trim and pretty good if I may so humbly say so!

A funny story proves that I definitely looked different and better from these changes (but they were not as easily done as what I will be explaining to you as the new lifestyle change I made at age 61 outlined in this book).

At SUNYA we were in suites of 3 rooms, two to a room and 6 in the suite. My senior roommate was a friend I had known for all four of my college years: Don Oppedisano. One of the suitemates was a guy named Walter Dreschler. We were going to see him the summer of 1969, just a year after our graduation and one year after our being suitemates also. Walt knew that Don was coming to Long Island to see him and he also knew that I would be accompanying Don, and he knew me very well also from my being in his suite for two years. We approached him on a sidewalk near his housing complex. He was talking only to Don and would occasionally look at me. I knew what was happening! He did not recognize me at all! But amazingly he said to Don after about 3-5 minutes "Well Don are you going to introduce me to this guy you brought with you and whatever happened to Rich anyways? I thought he was going to be with you?" Don was surprised and hadn't realized what was happening during his talk with Walt. When he told Walt that I was Rich, Walt was shocked out of his mind and raved. When we entered his house he yelled to his wife "You've got to come out here and see Rich! You won't recognize him!" I had known his girlfriend, now his wife, also at the university.

I tell this story because this was a dramatic change in my look too-as dramatic as my recent change in look is also, but it was VERY much more difficult and time-consuming than what I did to get my change now. But both amounted to the same amazing conclusion!

Then in my twenties, I continued running an hour every day. Then something dramatic happened also. I developed a running injury and knew that I wouldn't be able to run for about two weeks. So I started to do weight training to stay in shape. When the two weeks for the injury to subside were over, I decided I would continue with the weight-training since I had developed my own weight-training program which I liked and had created myself. Mind you, I never have used free weights but always used machines. First it was Universal, then Nautilus, Cybex, Soloflex, and now Bowflex and Nautilus. I have used weight-training on machines now for probably 40 years.

When doing weight training you see yourself every day in the mirror and don't really see any change. It is the same as when you look at yourself in a mirror, you don't think you look older! But after doing the weight-training for about a year people were starting to say to me, "Hey you are looking really good-you must be working out hard". So it was starting to show in my body and now my chest was developing nicely. So since age 30 or so I have always had a very big and impressive chest.

I was also becoming a very successful cross country coach of long distance runners. So successful that I was offered and became the cross country/track coach at Marist College in Poughkeepsie, New York. I did this for 8 years in the 1970s and then 4 years in the late 1980s. But now I realize that I was helping all those young men develop problems with their hips, back, and knees which would plague them in later life! Running is a bad way to do cardio. In a later chapter here I will outline the only three good ways to do cardio and go into detail on the one I specialize in now= walking!

So just before I started on my "lifestyle change" in 2007, I would get complements on my body all the time. I had a good looking chest and body. But I realized that I was 5-15 pounds overweight and especially around my stomach area= those terrible love handles we develop as men in later life!

So I tried everything I could to rid myself of those excess 5-15 pounds. Included in that list of things were special supplements, pills, and diets. It was the stomach and love handles section which were my trouble areas.

So now you can see that throughout all my life I have been concerned about my "over-weightness" and tried everything I could to develope a better weight. But sometimes the easiest thing is the last thing you try and you find out it is the best thing too!

# CHAPTER 3

## "Diets" In General...Why They Fail!

There are so many diets out there. Why? Because they all fail and are only successful for a short period of time. Many have been hailed as the greatest thing. What happens is you go on these diets and you are excited for a bit of time. You do lose some weight, but then the excitement goes away or you miss some of the foods you used to love but can't eat in this new special diet. Then you start little by little chipping away and doing things not in the diet plan and slowly you go back to the weight you were when you started your diet, or even more than that weight. You have spent a lot of money and wasted time on this temporary fix.

Also these diets are not nutritious and are boring. They cause you to lack certain important food group elements and are not healthy. You do not get a balanced menu of food groups. You even lose motivation after a while. You are not eating the kinds of foods you crave and want. You are told what to eat, when to eat it, and even how much of it to eat. This is fine with you when you start, but not for the rest of your entire life. This type of plan usually lasts anywhere from one to six months and then you go off it completely and try something new.

Some experts or companies talk about food items which make you get filled up or "satisfied" quicker. I tried these diets and actually ate more than when I didn't use them. Many "diet" foods actually have things in them to make you addictive to eating more of other things and the company gets richer even more quickly. Never eat anything that has a label "diet" on it. The plan outlined here does not want you to eat anything that says 'diet" or "fat free" or any of those kinds of terms.

There was even a study done with two groups. One group drank diet soda, the other regular soda. They were both given the same other kinds of foods to eat as a buffet where they could eat as much as they wanted. The group drinking the diet soda gained more weight than the non-diet soda group! The reason was that the diet soda had additives in it that made you addictive to eating even more of other foods. Companies know this and do it on purpose so you eat and buy more foods!

You will find the new "diet" or "lifestyle" plan outlined in this book to be tremendously easy. It will work and you will eat less and be healthier than ever! And you will never want to leave the plan and will use it the rest of your long life!

# CHAPTER 4

## Why This Diet Will Work-It's a new Lifestyle! It's So Easy-Eat Anything You Want!

The reason why this diet works and will work for you as much as it worked for me is that it is not really a "diet". It is better termed a "life-style". And you can eat anything and everything you want: Just as long as you can find that food item in the same classification as the main ingredient that this lifestyle asks for! You will not be missing any foods that you like. I love ice cream and I have ice cream every day. I even bought and use an ice cream maker and sometimes even make my own ice cream. But I also buy ice cream brands adherent to the goals of this program. I eat cakes, cookies, candies, pasta, pizza, and potatoes. I eat all kinds of carbohydrates: starches and sugars. I do not keep track of the amount of calories or carbohydrates or fats I eat each day or meal. You can do this and I provide you with guides/planners/charts you can use to help you if you are so-motivated to do so. But it is not necessary. You will be filled up quicker than any other diet you have ever tried! You will not be missing any food groups or foods you particularly enjoy eating. That is self-motivation right there! And it is proven to work...I know. All else failed, but it worked for me and I have remained at my same weight and looks now for over 3 years of being on this "diet". I have even lost a few more pounds in the last year (see Epilogue). I do not want to go off this diet and I never will. Why would I? I eat anything and everything I want to eat, have received the most complements from so many people, and I am the healthiest and happiest of my entire life. I am in the best shape and looks of my life and the best health of my life. And it is unbelievably easy. So why would I ever want to go off this new lifestyle? And the foods are the tastiest I have ever eaten too!

The secret with this lifestyle is that all the foods you eat have no additives or preservatives in them to make you addictive to eating more than you should eat or need to eat. You will be filled and "satisfied" quicker.

All the tips given here will help you reach your life-long weight/looks/health/goals!

# CHAPTER 5

## What I've Accomplished- Beyond My Wildest Dreams/Expectations!

When I started on this "lifestyle" in 2007 I merely wanted to lose maybe 5-15 pounds at the most and reduce my "love handles". I never ever dreamed or expected what would happen to me. That is why I have no "before" pictures to show you! I do not even remember when I started using a scale and started to notice the changes happening. They happened the right way...gradually and continuously. And I have maintained all the good statistics. The changes were accomplished in about 4-5 months of time.

Here are the amazing statistics:

BEFORE: 215#, 34" waist, with some "love handles"

AFTER: 185#, 30" waist, virtually NO "love handles"

For those of you who are weak in math, that means I lost 30 pounds and 4 inches off the waist and lost the love handles. All of this was accomplished easily in just 4-5 months of time! That is a safe loss of 13.5% of weight in 4-5 months of time or about 1/4 of a pound a day, or 1.5-2 pounds a week=all safe increments. It is for this reason that I also ask you NOT to weigh yourself for the first month and then only at most once a week after that! You do not want to lose a lot of weight too quickly...you want a gradual but continuous safe weight loss.

But those statistics are not the ONLY thing that changed. Here are more remarkable things that happened from this lifestyle change.

CHOLESTEROL:
BEFORE: 229

AFTER: 175 with both the good and bad types of cholesterol in the good normal range

TRIGLYCERIDES:
BEFORE: 140

AFTER: a mere 50!! (This is excellent since they are supposed to be under 150!!)

BLOOD PRESSURE:
BEFORE: I had slightly high blood pressure; so much on the high side that the doctor had me on one high blood pressure medication pill each night.

AFTER: I no longer have high blood pressure with my pressure readings at normal range and I am off the medication pill completely!

I am taking absolutely no medication pills of any kind and have excellent health. I do not get colds or any sicknesses. I think I might have been getting or had a cold once in the winter of 2009. But if it was a cold, it was over in 2-3 days and I hardly noticed it at all. It was so miniscule that I do not even know if I had a cold then! And I work teaching high school and college students who are constantly sick with colds, coughing, and sneezing in the classroom near me, and they have flus and other sicknesses too.

Again it was after this lifestyle change that a man said "You have the body of a 20-year old!" People usually guess that I am 37-52 years old. That means that I LOOK 10-25 years younger than my actual age number. I also did something I did not think possible: got rid of my "love handles"!
I am not sure if it will help your facial "looks', but most think my face is quite younger looking than my age number and I do not have wrinkles…just some forehead lines.

My weight is staying within 3 pounds of what seems like my "ideal" weight of 185 pounds.

I always seem to be anywhere from 182 to 188 pounds when I do my weekly weight check. And I have been at this same range all 3 years of my lifestyle change. Now as noted in the Epilogue I am even slightly less in weight at around the 170-175 mark.

I always kid others and say "I am not in the top 5% of the best bodies in the world, but I MIGHT be (and I say MIGHT as I am a humble and modest kind of guy!) in the top 5% of the best bodies of 64-year old guys!

Again all this was accomplished by making this one simple, easy-to-do lifestyle change and I never ever dreamed or expected all of this would happen. I would have been happy with just a 5-15 pound weight loss, but this is unbelievable and it was soooooooooo easy. And why would I or anyone else want to go away from it when it is so easy and so good!! And I won't go away from it ever!

# CHAPTER 6

# What You Will Accomplish

It is good to know ahead of time exactly what you will accomplish if you follow the plan as outlined in this book. And I make these as <u>GUARANTEES</u> IF you follow the plan as outlined here. And again it is a SIMPLE plan to follow and one you will want to follow and you will have no trouble following.

Some books/authors claim you will lose a certain amount of weight poundage. That is ridiculous! One Diet I once tried said that if you follow it, you would lose 20 pounds in 20 days. So let me get this right; a person weighing 500 pounds will lose just 20 pounds (4% of his/her body weight) while another person weighing just 100 pounds when they start that diet will also lose 20 pounds (20% of his/her body weight)? It should be a case that you will lose a PERCENTAGE of your total body weight.

Here are those <u>GUARANTEES</u> that will happen to you if you follow the plan of this book to the fullest:

1) I profess that you will lose anywhere from 10-20% of your body weight within 3-6 months of your start. It depends on your individual body metabolism, how much you do weigh, and just how strictly you do follow the program outlined here. It will be a gradual but continuous and safe weight loss week by week = safe and healthy!

2) You will look better than you have in years-maybe the best of your life even! I am not guaranteeing that there will be changes in your FACE, but perhaps even that will look better. Isn't it amazing how often when men and women who were obese and lose hundreds

of pounds all of a sudden become handsome men or beautiful-looking women! So even that is possible with this program. But I am saying that your BODY will be the best looking it has been in many many years and perhaps, like me, the best in your entire life, even at an older age!!

3) You will get your cholesterol and blood pressure back to normal and healthy range!

4) You will be in much better health. The incidences of flu and colds will be minimal and you will be in the best health of your recent years and perhaps of your entire life also. I am on no medications of any kind now for instance and never get sick!

5) Others will wonder what you have done and they will notice visible changes in you!

6) Strangers who do not know your background will guess your age wrong= lower! Again most think I am anywhere from 10 to 25 years younger than my age, with the average guess being 15 years younger than my age. Most guess that I am in my 40s or early 50s!

7) You will definitely have higher self-esteem and be proud to wear those skimpy swim suits you wouldn't dare wear now!

8) You will stand up taller and prouder and never even think of leaving the new lifestyle "diet" you have started since the foods taste better, are better for you health-wise and you want to maintain or even improve more your new healthy and great look! You will be even more motivated to stay on the program!

9) You will not be afraid to be seen swimming, tanning, beaching, or working out in public.

10) You will accomplish all of the above with no sacrifices on things you love to eat. Again it is the Easiest Diet in the World. And It Works!

# CHAPTER 7

## This Diet/Lifestyle Is Now Revealed...Why/How To Do It!

<u>PART ONE= THE "DIET"= MAIN COMPONENT PART</u>

Ok so we've spent six chapters getting you all riled up and trying to show you that there is some "diet' out there that is sooooo easy to follow, that allows you to eat anything you want/like, and still you lose the pounds, look the best of your life, and get all kinds of complements Quite amazing boasts! So what is this "diet" or "lifestyle"?

There is only one "ingredient" to it. And that "ingredient" is <u>ORGANIC</u>. You just have to be sure that anything and everything you eat is <u>ORGANIC</u>. Preferably CERTIFIED ORGANIC.

But what exactly does ORGANIC mean?? Organic food is free of pesticide, chemical fertilizer, food coloring, genetic modifications, cloning, antibiotics, steroids, hormones, chemicals, preservatives, additives, and other unknown elements. The land on which the vegetables and fruit are grown, and the pasture on which the cattle graze, have been cleaned for a minimum of three years.

Therefore organic foods have no additives or preservatives in them that make you addictive to eating more than you want or need. Here's some reasoning. You know how Asians are so noted for eating their rice and being so thin over in The Far East. Well many of them move to the United States and after they move here to the United States of America still eat the same kinds of food items that they ate over in their native lands. But after only a few years those lean thin Asians are now typical overweight Americans. How come? It is because the American food companies have put additives and preservatives in those same food items they ate in the Far East. Thus they eat more and more than they want & should and they buy more of the companies' foods and the food companies get richer!

So it is simple. Just eat foods certified to be organic. They have no additives or preservatives in them. I eat any food I want. I can still remember my very first all-organic meal. To save from typing the word "organic" over and over again, just remember that everything I now tell you was all organic with all organic ingredients and condiments used. I started with a tossed salad of lettuce, herbs, tomatoes and salad dressing. I ate my usual portion, not realizing that it was filling me up more than the same amount of "non-organic" salad would have. Then I put the same amount of pasta I would regularly have put on my plate. I was amazed that I could only eat about 1/3 of it! One-third of the amount I would have normally eaten. I was literally stuffed! There were no additives or preservatives. And it tasted sooooooo good too. That was just the beginning of it all! Every meal was the same way. Every meal I could only eat about 1/3 to 1/2 of what I would have normally eaten of the non-organic variety. And it all tasted so good too!

I love ice cream and eat ice cream every day, but only about 1/3 to 1/2 of what I used to eat because I am filled up so much more quickly. It's not that I say to myself "Well I better stop eating this stuff or I will gain weight". I am just stuffed! It comes automatically and naturally to me! By the way the best organic ice cream I have found is Alden's Organic Ice Cream. They have these in great flavors too: cookies and cream, mint chocolate chip, chocolate chocolate chip, raspberry, and the usual vanilla bean. Try these and tell me that they aren't extremely tasty! And I eat pasta, potatoes, starches, sugars, candies, cakes, brownies, cookies...you name it...but ALL ORGANIC. They all taste so good and better even than their non-organic counterparts! I do not worry about the number of calories or the amount of carbohydrates or fats I am eating; but you could even monitor that and probably even reach your weight loss goals quicker or even better if you did keep track of those amounts. More about how to monitor your situation comes up later in this book though. I have some helpful advice, tips, and charts for you to use if you wish.

Also I drink nothing but natural spring water or organic fruit juices and drinks. All the meats I cook are organic with no hormones given to the animals and no preservatives or additives. The eggs are certified organic. They are from grass fed free-range chickens. Fish is never certified organic, but you can eat any fish you want...just try not to use breaded or fried fish much. All the raw fruits and vegetables I cook and eat are certified organic with no pesticides or preservatives used.

It is especially important that all packaged foods, frozen entrees, canned foods, meats, dairy products, and drinks should all be organic. You will not eat as much as you used to, and you will be amazed. The pounds will come off and you will still eat your favorite foods and drinks, just that they are certified organic.

There are also some great tasting organic snack-type bars too! Besides the strictly 100% organic bars are Cliff bars. These are very close to being all-organic and come in many varieties. Among them are the ones made with organic oats and soybeans (like Chocolate Chip Peanut Crunch), the Cliff Builder bars (natural protein bars), and the Cliff Kid Z bars (and the kid in me eats them and I don't care....maybe that is why I look so young!). Also Kashi makes Go Lean bars that are close to being organic with all natural ingredients (chocolate peanut, chocolate almond, and chocolate caramel).

Now before I started the diet change, I was already working out and already doing cardio stuff every day, so the ONLY change I made in my lifestyle was switching to all organic foods. So that is what made me lose 30 pounds, 4" off my waist, and those love handles. The ONLY change I made was switching my foods and drinks to all organic ones. So that HAD to be what lead to my reduced weight! It was so easy and it worked. It will work for you too for sure!

PART TWO= EASY/FUN CARDIO

Now just switching to an all-organic food diet is going to make it work for you, but I strongly recommend also doing cardio every day. And I have more about this coming up in more detail later in this book. I do one hour of safe, easy, and fun cardio each day without fail. In 2009 I only missed my one hour of cardio less than five times and it was because I was traveling and getting into a "strange" city late at night when it was dark. And hey, doing my cardio is a time for me to show off my new body and hear those cars honking and people's comments too! I will explain later the only three types of "safe" cardio to do and explain how to do the cardio so it is more fun and I give you many tips. It is EASY and fun and I would not think of cutting it out. It is a time for contemplation during my day and also exploration of wherever I am doing the cardio.

You can just start as I did with 10 minutes and then gradually add on five minutes per day until you achieve one continuous hour of cardio. I do my cardio in the form of walking and exploration of whatever area I happen to be located in that day and tie it in with my day's travels, obligations, and activities as I will explain later. I also reward myself during this hour walk as I will explain later.

## PART THREE= WEIGHT TRAINING COMPONENT

Now this third component, weight training, is the least important and you can achieve 80-90% or more of the success I did without doing it at all. But hey, I wouldn't get all those raves about my chest if I didn't do this part and it's good to hear those raves!

You start with low weights and many repetitions and gradually add on weight week by week or month by month. I only concentrate on two body parts: my strongest body part, my chest, and what I think is my weakest, my stomach. [Although as I said I even get "comps" on my stomach now too!] You can do things for your arms as well as your legs, but your legs will be improved by your hour of cardio each day anyway!

I add more tips on this third component, weight training, also later in this book and even recommend a few supplements I take which can only help if you take them regularly too.

# CHAPTER 8

# Oh No- The Only Difficult Thing!

Oh No-there is a Difficult Thing! No, nothing I have told you is false. It IS the Easiest Diet in the World and It DOES work! But there is one difficult thing. Well maybe two difficult things. But both of them can be corrected and I wrote this book in the hopes that by YOUR going onto this diet or lifestyle BOTH of the "difficult things' will be diminished a lot and improved. So what are they?

First, the cost of organic food is 3 or 4 times the cost of the same item if non-organically produced/purchased. However, since you are eating only 1/3 to 1/2 as much, then actually I figure that you will have to spend about twice as much on food costs as you currently do (so NOT 3 or 4 times as much as you currently do). It is well worth the added expense though! And what extra amount you spend on food costs, you will be spending a lot less on medical costs. Also you can eventually buy clothing that will last a lifetime, as your weight and size won't change after you get down to your "ideal" weight. Oh that is something else that I did not mention before. I figure also that the organic lifestyle will get you down to your own personal "ideal" weight eventually. For me I have found my ideal weight to be right around 185 pounds. It doesn't matter if I go on a cleansing special diet which I mention later here, I eventually settle back at or near the 185 pound mark. Now perhaps it seems to be around the 175 pound mark even! The organic lifestyle will get you right there after about a year's time too!

So WHY is the cost of organic foods so much more than the non-organic counterparts when they are not buying and using chemicals, preservatives. and additives? There are several reasons. First since there are no preservatives, the food items spoil quicker and a lot of them must be discarded and the food companies must make up for the loss in revenue for the discarded food items. Second, the companies (and also local farm growers) must pay for the certification of "organic" by special companies which certify the foods. This costs a lot of money. Third, they have to go through and do a lot of specialized things to get the foods to be organic and go through rigid performance tests to do so. Once at a local San Diego Farmers Market I asked the local farmer if the fruit I was going to buy from them was certified organic. They said no because they could not afford to pay for the certification process. But for all intents and purposes, it was organic. I bought the item! Fourth, the amount of people buying organic products is so much less than the non-organic varieties. Thus the more of you who start buying organic, the price will come down...see...my selfish reason for writing this book too!

The second difficult thing about this organic diet is that it is harder to find organic foods than regular foods I must admit. However with more and more people realizing the benefits of the all-organic diet (and especially with them reading and following the guidelines of this book and hearing my success story), more and more stores are selling organic products. Now you can find organic products in most major super market chains as well as specialty health-food type markets.

Now I have some ideas to help out with the first difficult thing mentioned here, the cost of organic foods. I do not believe that for the purposes of the weight loss goals that you will suffer much at all if you purchase non-organic raw fruits and vegetables instead of the certified organic raw fruits and veggies. So if you want to save a LOT of money you can simply purchase non-organic raw fruits and vegetables. But be sure that all canned, frozen, and packaged items as well as dairy and meat products are organic. I do not think this will affect your weight loss situation much, if at all, since the raw fruits and veggies do not have additives to make you addictive to eating more than you should eat.

Another way to save money is to first buy the organic food products at the major super market chains and especially in their own brand instead of the national brand names. You will also find that Costco is now selling a LOT of organic food items and at cheaper prices in the large bulk varieties.

Another way to save money (but you have to be VERY careful about this) is that some items not certified as "organic" are essentially organic foods. These food items are typically labeled "Natural" or "All Natural" or "Made with organic ingredients" (even though you will not see the special organic symbol which states the food item is certified organic). Look for this symbol. It is easy to spot. I can now spot it a mile away it seems! You have to be very careful though with these non-certified food items. Check the ingredients in them. If you cannot pronounce some of the ingredients, it means they are chemicals and not a good thing to be eating for your dietary purposes. But I have bought a lot of food items labeled as "natural" that are essentially organic foods that were simply not certified organic, but were organic for all intents and purposes. You can save a LOT of money when you buy these items! But again be very careful and try to limit the amount of these that you purchase also.

I find first of all that the food market which has the most quantity and also the most quality of organic products is Whole Foods Markets. Whole Foods Markets are found in many of the biggest cities in the United States and also in Canada as "Capers" Markets. However I find at Whole Foods that their own Whole Foods brand product line is very reasonably priced and even some of their non-certified organic products are essentially organic and are ok to purchase if you want to save money. I had some friends rave about Whole Foods' all organic double-creme oreo-type cookies-try these and tell me they aren't the best you ever ate! So the products there cost more than regular super market products because most of their products are indeed organic, which as we mentioned cost more than the non-organic food products of the same "type". It's like buying a Rolls Royce instead of buying a Ford!

Other big markets which sell large amounts of organic products include Henry's Markets, Trader Joe's, Nature's Best, and others across our country and world-wide. Look up on the internet under "organic food markets" and you will find stores near you. I have even found organic foods at dollar stores. One of the best dollar-type stores we have in the West are the 99 Cents Only stores. These are huge super-market size stores where everything is 99.99 cents or under. They have on occasion even had some organic items. Boy do I go crazy then!!! I remember one time when they had Organic Kraft Macaroni and Cheese packages at 3 for 99 cents! I bought 21 of them! Many times these stores get new samples of items to sell. So go crazy and stock up!

Again though it is worth the extra amount you will pay for the organic foods based on what is going to happen to your body, your health, your looks, and your weight!

# CHAPTER 9

## Where To Buy Foods/What To Get

In the last chapter I went into many details on ways to save money in the first of the two so-called "difficult" things about this lifestyle plan. They are difficult challenges, but BOTH are very reachable challenges as I have definitely accomplished overcoming (and very successfully so) both of these "obstacles".

Now in this chapter I am going to help you out in finding the organic foods. So I already explained how you should "hit the internet" and find which stores nearby have organic foods besides the obvious health-food markets and big chain supermarkets which carry many more organic food items than in the past. They will carry even more organic food items as more of you take on the organic food lifestyle suggested here. I find the toughest challenges for me are when I am traveling and vacationing. I was amazed that when I traveled to Orlando, Ft. Lauderdale, and St. Petersburg, Florida that there was a Whole Foods Market within a short distance of my hotel in each of those cities. Also it was even a short 5-10 minute walk when I visited those three great cities of the Northwest: Portland, Seattle, and Vancouver BC Canada on trips the last 2 summers. But I have several other tips and ideas I have successfully used even when away from home.

The first thing I try to do when I am traveling is to get a hotel room which has a small refrigerator and also a small microwave oven. Even if they do not have such items in the hotel's guest rooms, many will let you use the refrigerator in their employee's lounge or common-use continental breakfast room. If not, I have even gone on Craig's list and actually gone to a local person's house and purchased a small microwave for $10 for my 3-7 days stay in a town. I can usually get a small refrigerator for about $25. This is cheaper than some hotels which have cost me $10 extra per day for a refrigerator/microwave to be put in my room. But one hotel I stayed at even made sure that I had both of these items in my room when I registered a complaint that they had no common-use microwave for hotel guests in their facility. They did so at no additional charge and those two things were in my room upon my arrival. So don't give up and request/demand them! You will succeed! And with just those two items, you are all set to purchase and prepare breakfast, lunch, supper, and snack items that will keep you on the all-organic lifestyle. The small microwave is to heat up a frozen organic entree for supper use. But if you cannot get a microwave oven, the refrigerator will serve to satisfy your meal needs for the vacation. Recently I was on that 3-city vacation to Florida mentioned above and I would say I was able to eat organic foods 90-98% of the time! Some of the other items were all natural.

Make sure that the other products you buy are also organic: sea salt, spices, condiments (mayonnaise, ketchup, and mustard), spring water, and juices.

Now I did mention in an earlier chapter about a special diet I use once a year to cleanse out my body. It is something I have done now for the last 3 years and I strongly recommend it. It is obtainable from www.WholeFoodFarmacy.com or more information at 866-661-5011 or 507-726-4181. They are not affiliated with Whole Foods Market I found out. I go on this program every year after Thanksgiving and before Christmas for 13 days. You can choose a different time period if you like. I always lose a pound a day for the 13 days. I do regain the weight back slowly and gradually after I go back to my all-organic regular lifestyle, but the 13-day program totally detoxes me and cleanses me fully. That was another reason why I think my ideal weight is around the 185-pound mark after doing this special weight-loss/cleansing program the last 3 years and after losing 13 pounds each year. You see I still eventually settled back into the 185-pound mark in about a month's time after going to my regular all-organic lifestyle. This special program is called WholeFoodFarmacy's Tri-Decathlon Delux full body cleanse and weight loss program for 13 days. It provides you with all you need to eat and drink for the 13 days at a listed price of $149.95. If that sounds expensive, remember that is the ONLY cost you will have for ALL of your food and drink for the 2-week period, so a very reasonable total price for two weeks' time and not expensive at all. It amounts to less than $12 per day! All the food is either certified organic or essentially is organic, just not with the certification. The items include the delicious basic staple of the "diet": phi plus (7 bags). a mixture of organically-certified fruits and nuts in a delicious snackable bag. Also included are the tasty spicy veggielicious spice (3 bags), the tasty fruitalicious plus (3 bags), and the amazing "rolls royce" of the diet: tropiphi, unbelievably delicious! You also get a detoxphi to use each day and stardust2hydr8 to put into your spring water. I can't tell you how easy it is to stay on this "diet' for the 13 days and how healthy it is as well. You do not lose energy and you feel great. I highly recommend this as a detox/cleanse once a year. The items can also be used during the year as snack food items and they are truly delicious! The ONLY drawback of the 2-week program for me is that I do wish I could eat those holiday meals I observe at the Holiday parties I am attending at the time. But I pick out that particular time period for a definite purpose. I actually think although it is a tough time period to go on this special once-a -year "diet" that it is also then the best time to do this program. I avoid all those non-organic meals and snacks offered at this time of the year! They also have a 24-hour support line too at 507-726-4080.

# CHAPTER 10

## Suggestions/Tips/My Daily Meal Ideas & Places To Eat Out

To end the food part of the 3-component "new lifestyle toward the new you", I wanted to put in some finishing touches with suggestions and ideas to help you. First as mentioned earlier I feel strongly that you should not weigh yourself for the first month or, if possible, even wait until two months after you have started this program. After that initial "weighing- in" though, it will be important for you to weigh yourself every week at the same time and place, and using the same scale and also wearing the same kind of clothes. I recommend weighing yourself in the morning and also completely naked. I weigh myself every Monday morning first thing. You should notice on your first weighing after you initiated this program that you have lost roughly 1-3 pounds per week. It all depends on your metabolism, body frame, and how much weight you had when you began the program. Then after the initial weighing-in you should notice drops of approximately 1-3 pounds per week, dependent on those same things again. Eventually after 4-6 months you will probably be at your ideal weight and plateau. But continue weighing yourself every week at the same time, place, scale, and method. If your weight goes up, look at your food charts if you do those charts which I have made available for you to use here. In my case, I simply think about what I have had to eat the past week. When I notice my weight has gone up 2-4 pounds in the week, I then question what food item I ate in excess or what different item I added to my food diet. In some cases I remembered that I was drinking a LOT of organic fruit juices, so I cut down on that and replaced the fruit juices with spring water. In another case I was eating a quart of the organic ice cream each night. So I cut that down to a pint each night. Every time this happened the very next week I was back to my ideal weight and had lost the necessary 2-4 pounds I desired. You can do the same, and with the use of the eating logs I provide here, it will make your changes even easier to figure out.

Now I want to give you an idea of what I actually eat in a sample day. My typical breakfast consists of a full organic grapefruit (using organic blue agave or organic honey as a sweetener) plus a supplement that I highly recommend called D4 Thermal Shock from Cellucor. Follow the directions carefully on the product. They tell you to start with just one capsule twice a day for about a week and then gradually increase it to 2 capsules twice a day. You will really feel it when you start taking these and won't want to take more than the prescribed amount! They attack deep fat deposits, skyrocket caloric burn, provide explosive energy, and help suppress appetite. I strongly recommend this supplement. It has proved very effective to me also. I have the grapefruit each breakfast because it has a special kind of acid in it that also helps you reduce weight. As long as you are not allergic to grapefruit, I strongly recommend one full grapefruit every breakfast. You remember the famous grapefruit diet…well that's why it worked! Then I add to these two staples for breakfast, something else. It could be 2-3 organic free-range eggs, 2 pieces of organic toast with even peanut butter and jelly on them (organic of course), or a special organic breakfast bar. I even sometimes have 5-10 chocolate chip cookies as my other item to have! I also at times have a big bowl of organic cereal with soy or organic milk.

For a mid-morning snack I have an organic bar with something to drink or cookies. The other snack time is when I do my one-hour walk (mid-morning or mid-afternoon usually) and with that I have a huge organic apple as I start my walk along with my spring water bottle. Wait till you taste organic fruit!

My typical lunch consists of a drink, organic yogurt (I love Wallaby's Maple yogurt as my #1 favorite brand and flavor), a pear, grapes or raisins, string cheese, and an organic bar. Sometimes (like today for instance) I had an organic sandwich on a hamburger-type roll with lettuce, tomatoes, cheese, turkey and mayo. Of course you know ALL of the ingredients were organic! I have increased the amount of fruit I eat since going all-organic and find organic fruits to be much better in taste and also fill you up better of course than the non-organic varieties I had eaten all of my previous years.

My supper consists of a salad with many different varieties of dressings. Whole Foods has a tremendous and very reasonably-priced light ranch salad dressing that I particularly enjoy. Then besides that I have perhaps chicken breasts cooked in various ways or pasta with meat balls or grilled hamburgers or even frozen entrees from companies. Again fish can be used too. Just avoid breaded fish or fried fish too much. My specialties that I make myself are my organic lasagna (vegetarian or with meat), shepherd's pie, and meat loaf. Everyone raves about these specialties of mine. I never used to cook much, but now I enjoy cooking, especially these specialties of mine! Or how about my grilled cheese meat loaf sandwich!

One of the best items I have ever tasted in the long list of great-tasting organic foods is organic bacon! As a matter of fact I was not offended at all when I had my friend Paul Gustafson for a week and had made my special organic shepherd's pie and also an organic meat loaf and asked him then at the end of his stay which food item was the best tasting of all. He said that although he loved my two specialties I had served him, the very best organic food he had tasted the whole week was the organic bacon. I am not talking here about turkey bacon, but actual pork organic bacon and it is tremendous and all the fat becomes non-fat under proper heating time too.

One "mistake" I did once is now something I feature in my meat lasagna. I wanted to add some sausage, but the only kind of sausage that I had in the house was breakfast apricot sausage. I know, it doesn't sound very appealing in meat lasagna. But boy did it give it tremendous taste and full flavor and now I purposely use it all the time on my meat lasagna!

As far as restaurants that I have discovered with organic dishes, there is a pizza chain that we have in San Diego and is also elsewhere in the country called Pizza Fusion. I recommend their all organic crusted pizza. In Los Angeles' West Hollywood section, I strongly recommend the best organic fast-food place I have ever had the pleasure to dine. It is called O! Burger featuring all organic hamburgers (meat, chicken, or veggie-your choice), plus the best organic French fries I have ever had and salad bowls and hot dogs, As they say in their place "If it's edible, it's organic!" They are located at 8593 Santa Monica Blvd. in West Hollywood. Tell co-owners Martha Chang and Andy Soboil that you read my book and raves about their place!

For great-tasting sandwiches, I go to Whole Foods Markets where you can tell them exactly what ingredients and type of bread you want them to put into your individually-prepared sandwiches. It will be one of the best sandwiches you ever had, and in the words of Richard Nixon, "Trust Me"! But this time it is true! Also when I am vacationing I also go into their stores. They have a microwave you can use and a cafeteria. I go to the frozen entrée section and select an organic frozen entre (lasagna, macaroni and cheese, etc.) and then heat it up in their microwave and eat it there in the cafeteria. I complete my meal with a pint package of organic ice cream from the freezer section too!

I had the pleasure recently while on vacation in Florida near Cocoa Beach and Merrit Island of eating at another organic restaurant that was fantastic. It is called "The Jungle Restaurant and Market". It is located at 2500 N Highway A1A in Indialantic FL. Their chefs use only the finest quality of organic ingredients. I particularly liked their pizza, jungle burger, and desserts as well as the selection of soups (they have 3 daily soups).

On a trip to New Hope Pennsylvania in August of 2010 I had the task of trying to find some restaurant in this small but quaint town which would have either fish that I liked or Thai food (which I find is CLOSE to being organic). Or of course could I possibly find any organic food in ANY restaurant in this small town? After looking up and down the main street of the town and not finding anything to my liking, I hit the jackpot! Just as I was ready to give up, I saw one place's menu on display. One of its specials was "organic chicken breast with organic baby vegetables and grits." Wow! I ate there twice! The grits are not organic, but they replaced that with a double order of the organic baby vegetables. The place is Martine's Riverfront Restaurant on East Ferry Street in New Hope. They are located right on the Delaware riverfront with both indoor and outdoor seating. I had a very good chat too with the waitress there about my book which was in the closing stages at the time and she also couldn't believe how OLD I was!!

These are just some of the organic restaurants that I have found to be excellent in my travels. Please tell me more when you come across others. You can email me at: TheEasiestDiet@ aol.com with your reviews of them! I want to include in the sequel to this book a complete listing of restaurants around the country and world which serve some organic food items.

By the way I have not received any promotional consideration payments from mentioning any of the above places or any products mentioned in this book.

# CHAPTER 11

## Only Three "Safe" Cardios

As I mentioned earlier, I use to run one hour straight (well sometimes on curved, jagged paths actually) since I graduated from SUNYA back in 1968. Then after doing that for about 30 years I had to stop running because my right knee hurt a lot. I went to my regular doctor and he took x-rays of the right knee and it showed nothing wrong. So he sent me to an orthopedic specialist who yanked me on a table and had me raise my legs up and he exclaimed "I don't think you have a knee problem. I think you have a right hip problem"! So he took x-rays of the right hip and it showed big-time arthritis of the cartilage there. He said "Some day you will need total right hip replacement surgery! Not now, but some day".

So I stopped running and pretty much did no cardio at all. That caused me to become even more slightly overweight. More on that later. When I moved to San Diego in 2001 the hip pain was getting worse, but still I did nothing about it except taking herbal supplements. Finally in 2007 I went to a free clinic put on by two orthopedic surgeons. One of them was Dr. Louis Levy who did his practice in nearby La Mesa, California, a suburb of San Diego. He was one of the top knee and hip replacement surgeons in the area and did his procedures at Sharp Grossmont Hospital also in La Mesa. He asked the audience to answer five questions and based on my answers to those 5 questions, it showed that I did not need the hip replacement surgery yet. (The questions were things like whether I avoided going to a friend's house that had a lot of steps to climb, etc.)

But wouldn't you know it! Within a month of attending that clinic, my pain got worse. I scheduled an appointment with Dr. Levy and it was probably three weeks before I could even see the busy surgeon. When I did get an appointment and spoke with him, he still did not pressure me about having the surgery but said it was my decision. I knew it was time. So On Oct. 2, 2007 I had my right hip replaced and Dr. Levy did a tremendous minimally-evasive procedure. I set records for being released from the hospital in just two days and never using a walker. I used two crutches. On the third day (I did NOT arise from the dead!) I used just one crutch. On the fourth day after surgery I was walking with just the use of a cain. And after only five days from the surgery I was able to walk without the aid of anything but my own two feet. I then started doing daily ten-minute walks and increased the time about 5 minutes per day until after about two weeks from the surgery date I was walking an hour straight every day. And I have continued to do so ever since! Dr. Levy says that I could run if I wanted to. But if I did, I would need that hip replacement done again to my right hip in 10-15 years. If I simply do the only 3 safe types of cardio, I would never need that hip redone again, barring any unforeseen problems or a new injury such as a fall down stairs.

Dr. Levy was himself a runner. I was a coach of high school and college distance runners in cross country and track. Running is a good cardio exercise to do. But our bodies are not made for the constant hard jarring and high impact of running. The ONLY 3 safe cardio exercises to do are walking, swimming, and bicycling. Since I am a spastic bicyclist and I do not have a swimming pool, walking was the one for me! The high impact of running is detrimental to five areas: your two hips, your two knees, and your back area. I think now of all of those distance runners I coached through the years and who continued to run after they graduated and how they are probably going to need major surgery on their knees, hips, or back some time in their life.

So I will tell you how I have developed a fun, easy, safe, and rewarding walking program to add to your organic diet lifestyle. This program will improve your health, especially heart, pulse, cholesterol, and blood pressure as well as it will help in keeping your weight down and also be motivational and fun!

# CHAPTER 12

## How To Do The Walking and Have It Be Fun!

I have a friend who does his cardio in the form of a walk every day. Good. But he does the same exact path every day...wow! How boring! I couldn't do that...actually I should say that I wouldn't want to do that! I walk one hour every day, but try to use a variety of different places. Hey, variety is the spice of life! This makes it more fun, motivational, and I incorporate exploration into it too. I have actually even found new routes of travel for me to use in my car in case of traffic problems!

So first of all I have told you that I choose walking as my "safe" cardio to use every day. It was one of those three "safe" cardios that Dr. Levy told me about and I explained in the last chapter. But I have a LOT of advice and suggestions here in this chapter to make your walk rewarding and more fun. My one-hour walking routine is just a matter of setting aside the time to do it now. I missed less than five days of walking in the year 2009 and that was due to my travel schedule and not being able to get out and do it because of arriving in the dark in a strange city.

First I try to incorporate my walk in my regular day's schedule. For instance, if I am going to go to the bank and drive there, I do it from there. If I am going to a supermarket, I do it from there. If I am going to the mall, I do it from there. In general, what I do is I walk from my car a half hour and then turn around and walk back to my car. I can also tell from this method how my second half pace is compared to my first half. Sometimes I have an extra minute or two to do at the end to complete the one hour I want to walk. That means my second half was even faster in pace than my first half. Sometimes I actually do not reach my car when the hour is already up. That means my second half was slower than my first half.

The hardest place to walk is in a big city. And the hardest intersection to encounter in a city is at a busy traffic light. However you can always go in one direction there. So in a city I do what I call "hap-hazard" walks. That means that I select two general directions and whenever I get to a traffic light, I go in either one of those two directions. For instance I could pick North and East, or North and West, or South and East, or South and West. Then if I chose North and East as my two-directional option for example, when I get to a light I go either North or East there, depending on which way the light allows me to travel. I continue this trend all the time for the first half of the walk, but then on the way back I might be doing a different route than my first half depending on what traffic light situations I encounter. But I will make it back to my car by now going South and West all the time at each traffic light intersection I encounter. I find these "hap-hazard" routes the best way to handle city streets. The key thing is: never stop walking...always keep moving. The best thing that you can encounter is a 4-way stop for traffic where cars must stop in all four directions at that intersection. Then you can definitely continue in the same direction you want to go for sure. The worst things to encounter are those busy hectic traffic lights. But the "hap-hazard" idea that I explained here works for the traffic lights, or else I just walk around the sidewalk near the light until the light changes for me to move onward.

Another motivational thing I do for my daily walks is that I reward myself for doing them. When I start out on my walk, I eat my apple for the day. This is my reward. I also carry with me a small bottle of water to drink as I go along. This has proved very valuable too for "emergency" type situations. One time while on vacation in Chicago I tripped and fell down because of an uneven pavement on the sidewalk. You Chicagoans must improve your sidewalks!! Luckily, I was not too badly hurt, but had some cuts. I used the water in the bottle to help my recovery from those cuts and thus it helped me out a lot. Also sometimes the apple's skin gets stuck in my mouth and I have used the water to get the apple skin swallowed down my throat better. So besides the obvious need of water, especially in warm weather, it can really help you out in emergency-type situations too. So I suggest carrying a water bottle and also some reward such as the apple or a pear or something to reward yourself for the daily walk. I also carry my personal ID card and a cell phone during the walks too of course. And a handkerchief also helps in sweat-weather conditions and for other uses too. So to summarize, the things I bring on my walk again are: ID, cell phone, handkerchief, reward (apple), and water bottle.

So my former one-hour runs that I used to do before my hip replacement surgery, have now become daily one-hour walks. I have about ten "paths' I do from my own house. Even varying the direction of some of the loops I have makes them different. But again I also try to incorporate my walk on my daily schedule and after I park my car, I just go out one-half hour from my car and then come back to my car. This is the method I try doing the most, especially when vacationing or when traveling to a new place.

It is amazing to me how in a strange city I have even found very safe and interesting walks by some miracle. I hardly ever, if ever, have been on a dangerous walk where you run into high traffic or busy intersections or freeways. Again in a city I use the "haphazard" method explained above to handle that and I have used that often too in my own downtown San Diego. I have done successful walks in Los Angles, Portland, Seattle, Vancouver BC Canada, Houston, Orlando, Fort Lauderdale, and St. Petersburg as well as Tijuana and Puerto Vallarta in Mexico.

# CHAPTER 13

## Other Ideas on Cardio

We have gone over the 3 "safe" cardios and some recommended ways to successfully accomplish the cardio segment of your new lifestyle in doing your hourly daily walk. I have some additional ideas on cardio to help you.

First it is very good to add stretching and flexibility if you can. Yoga is excellent too.

As far as machines for cardio, a tread mill utilizes too much stress and impact on your hips, back, and knees. It is the same "bad" cardio as running unless you use it just for walking. And if you do that, you might as well go outside and do your walks...much more interesting and motivational! However there are two good cardio machines. One is a mountain-climbing machine. Another which I recommend and use a lot is the Precor Elliptic Cross Trainer. This simulates walking/running with no impact on your body parts. It is very useful to use. However it is not as motivational or exciting as walking. I also use my walking time as a time for me to think about the day's schedule of other activities and things I must do.

There is another thing I have done when I was injured and therefore not able to run back in those days when I was running. This could still be done instead of walking when you can't walk due to a foot or leg injury. What I would do then and now you could also do to replace your daily walk when you are injured is to take exercises that you can do and do them continuously for an hour. Do situps, pushups, chinups, and any other exercises and just do them continuously for an hour's worth of time. Obviously this is not as exciting or motivational as walking in exciting pathways in your community. So I would only think of doing this if I had an injury and could not actually walk.

It is hard to impossible to walk at an airport or some other places where you are waiting around and have nothing else to do. The crowds and people around make it virtually impossible and your pace would have to be very slow also.

The key thing in your cardio is to keep moving for an hour continuously. And remember if you can't do one hour of continuous movement when you begin your new lifestyle program, start with five minutes and gradually increase the time each day until you can do a continuous hour.

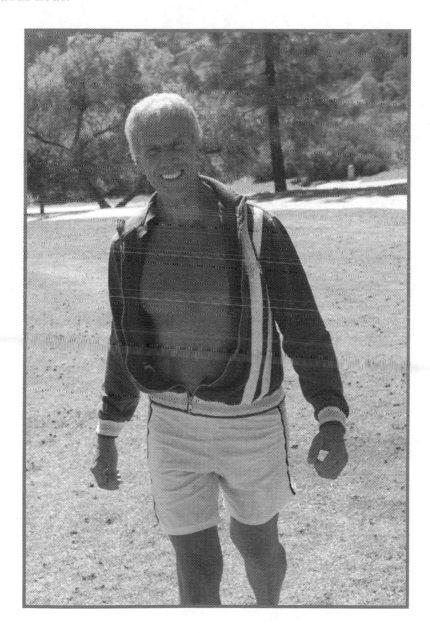

# CHAPTER 14

## Supplements You Can Take

Although it is not necessary to take ANY supplements with the new lifestyle change you will be utilizing, I can suggest some here that work nicely and can also benefit you. I have already mentioned the D4 Thermal Shock capsules I take twice a day from Cellucor. They definitely help me in attacking fat deposits and, as I said before, when you start taking them you KNOW they are working! You can feel the effects. Be sure to consult your physician of course before starting any new dietary program such as this (although this new lifestyle program is based on eating healthy organic foods and definitely should not cause any hardships as long as you are not allergic to certain food items and therefore still do not eat those food items even organically). But consult your physician and also follow the directions on the dietary supplements carefully before taking any of these supplements that I am recommending here.

Just before I do my weight training workouts and also during the workout I also take GNC's Advanced Muscle Performance Amplified N.O. Loaded. It has a micronized nitric oxide formula. It helps to volumize muscle cells and improves strength. It is absorbed rapidly in the body and generates an increase in muscle power. I definitely feel it has maximized the benefits of my weight training efforts.

You can ask the workers at GNC about this product or other products you can take as supplements. I trust their knowledge and expertise. I feel that the supplements you can take should be to maximize the benefits of your weight training and/or to cut down on fat deposits you may have in your body.

Another thing I take is for my own sun tanning. I try to use tanning products which have caffeine in them as it has been shown in some studies that caffeine helps to prevent skin cancer. I use a really fine product I get from Hawaii and people rave about my good natural dark tan color. It is called Maui Babe Browning Lotion. Be careful as it has no SPF. But some say that it is the chemicals from the SPF ingredients that actually cause skin cancers! Another thing I have heard which also makes sense is that if you wouldn't drink or eat a particular product, you should not apply that product to any part of your skin. Your skin is an organ and all the stuff you put onto your skin is going to seep into your body. So if you wouldn't drink that product or eat it, why would you want to put it into your body via your skin? This sun tanning browning lotion contains actual coffee plant extract (you can smell it when you apply it to your skin) and is all natural in its ingredients. There have been some studies which have concluded that caffeine helps to prevent skin cancers, although the results in other such studies have proved inconclusive. However this product definitely produces for me a fast and very dark tan and it MIGHT be helping to prevent skin cancer too! You could order some by calling them at 1-800-250-3581.

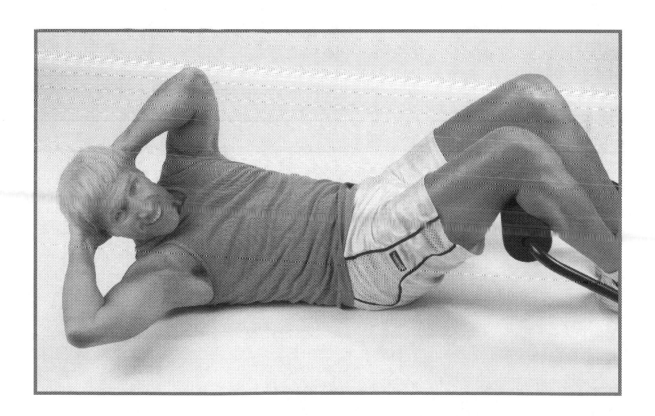

# CHAPTER 15

## Weight Training Ideas If You Want to
## Add This "Finishing Touch

I have spent the most time here talking about the two most important components of the new lifestyle of the new YOU! Those two most important items are the diet component and then, less important than that, the cardio component. The "finishing touch" or third component and definitely the least important of the three is weight training. If you can add this one, great. If you can't or don't wish to add it, you will still do extremely well and reduce a lot of weight by following the dietary component and even more if you add the cardio component as well.

I also make this component as much fun as possible. Thus many people are surprised when they learn that I have never ever used free weights in my weight training routine... I have only used machines of different kinds. First it was Universal, then Soloflex, then Nautilus, then Cybex, and now Bowflex. They are safer than using free weights and you can move more quickly thru the exercises and they also are more fun. There is no question though that you can make even bigger gains and make those gains faster if you use free weights. But to me, the advantages of using machines far outweigh the added muscular advantage of using free weights.

I am currently using the newest Bowflex machine called the Bowflex Revolution. It is the nearest thing to free weights that I have ever seen or used and is used by NASA in the training of its astronauts. It is safe, fun, and very effective. It simulates a LOT of the benefits derived from the use of free weights. I just concentrate on my upper body and particularly my chest. I also do exercises using a thera crunch machine for my abs. So that is all I do: chest and abs. My strongest point (chest) and my weakest point in looks (abs).

However I have gotten so many more complements on my chest now even though I believe it is only minutely bigger than it used to be. That is because my waist is now 30" and not 34", so my chest looks even bigger with the smaller waist size protruding! As I mentioned earlier in this book I have even gotten some complements in the last year about my stomach! Wow!

I recommend starting out with low weight and doing many repetitions and then gradually adding on the weight. I now do 3 sets of 73 reps each of butterfly or pec dec exercise for my chest and then 3 sets of 73 reps each of incline chest press for my chest. I do 6 sets of 73 reps of abs exercises. I also start my weight training by doing one set of 73 reps of a rowing type exercise as a sort of warm-up to loosen up my upper body in preparation for the upcoming chest exercises. The number "73" is not my lucky number. I have advanced to this number through the years, but I started with a much smaller number of repetitions: probably started with 20 or so. The whole weight training workout takes about one hour and in-between sets I do things around the house that need to get done. I have the advantage of having a home gym outside on my side porch with a roof over it. I do the weight training every other day which is what you should do to allow your muscles to grow between workout days. You do not need to do any kind of weight training for your legs as your legs will receive all the benefits they need during your daily cardio exercise.

## A TYPICAL DAY OF MY WEIGHT-TRAINING PROGRAM

1) One set of 73 reps of rowing exercise and then a set of 73 reps of thera crunch abs exercise; then rest 2-3 minutes
2) I then alternate a set of 73 reps of pec dec or butterfly chest exercise with a set of 73 reps of thera crunch abs exercise, doing a total of 3 sets of each; first a pec dec set followed by abs crunch set and resting 2-3 minutes after doing the abs exercises.
3) I end by alternately doing a set of 73 incline chest presses with a set of 73 reps of thera crunch abs exercises and again doing a total of 3 sets of each: first the incline chest press followed by abs crunches and resting again 2-3 minutes after doing the abs exercises.
I increase the poundage on the weight exercises after doing them for a few weeks and being able to easily accomplish the workout.

# CHAPTER 16

## Epilogue

It has now been three years that I have maintained this new lifestyle. It has also now been about nine months since I began writing this book. And I can't believe it, but I have been doing the all-organic 'diet" now for three years...doesn't seem possible and I will continue it the rest of my life for sure!

Complements keep coming as I meet strangers and even old friends who have not seen me for many years. They are all amazed and the complements give me even more confidence and reason to stand up prouder and taller.

Here is just one sample of the TYPE of thing I get. On a particular website that has a small photo of me and my age on it, I got a response from someone in Aug. of 2010, and I asked them why they had even bothered looking at my profile at all. They responded, "cause I was trippin on your age and how good you looked for your age. I think it's really cool that you're keeping yourself together—you're an inspiration! You look great!" I get these kind of remarks all the time now!

My weight is now even slightly less than the 185 I thought was my "ideal" weight. I am now centered about the 175-180 range and it has been as low as 172 and never higher than 181 in the last 3-4 months. Just remember that toned muscle tissue weighs more than the same mass of fat.

Also over the summer of 2010, I visited the Northeast area of the United States, in particular Ogunquit Maine, the Hudson Valley of New York State, and New Hope, Pennsylvania. I heard stories of three other people who also went all-organic and they also lost a LOT of weight. So this inspired me more and convinced me that I was not just a special case of this affect. It showed me that if anyone went all-organic in their food and drink intake, they also could lose weight and easily so.

For a last example, just a week before this book was sent to the publisher, I was celebrating its purported successful completion in a Labor Day weekend vacation trip to Laguna Beach. I first went to the beach and then went to checkin at my hotel. I entered the hotel lobby with no shirt and just short shorts on. The manager of the hotel came up to me and said something like "Well how long do you workout every day to look like that!" I told him only about 15-30 minutes every other day and an hour walk every day. He was amazed. I told him how it was more about my diet. I asked him to guess how old I was. He looked me over carefully and said "Around 45!" I said that was about the average guess and then floored him with my age of 64. So it just keeps on amazing people and keeps on looking and feeling good for me!!

This idea is a completely new idea or reason for someone to eat organic foods. In the past people touted organic foods for environmental reasons or because it tasted better or because it was healthier. While these are all still true and great reasons to consume organic foods, this dietary reason is revolutionary but is logically deduced from my own experience sited in this book. With all the chemical ingredients added to our foods, these preservatives and additives only tend to diminish the food's natural nutrients. They also cause addiction for you to want to eat more. It is like those who add salt or oils to foods also.

NOTE: For the record, for my last "weigh-in" before I sent this manuscript to the publishers in September of 2010, I was now at 172 pounds and I have been holding very closely there for the last month!

# CHAPTER 17

## Sequel To This Book

I have already established and imagineered a sequel to this book. It is going to be called "The Easiest Diet in the World… How It Has Worked For EVERYONE Who's Followed It!"

You will be the writers of this book. You will send me the material to be published in it. If you follow this book's program, whether just the dietary concerns and/or you also include the cardio and/or weight-training aspects of it too, I want to hear your stories. Send me the following:

1) Your before and after photos.
2) Your before and after measurements and statistics.
3) Tell me the time elapsed from the start of the program to the end of it, i.e. whether it is four, five, or six months.
4) Tell your amazing entire story!

Email any or all of the above four items to: TheEasiestDiet@aol.com

Some may think that this book is egotistical on my part. Well the ONLY way I could convince you of what this new lifestyle can do for you was through my own experience. There haven't been any completed research studies yet on the effects of organic food consumption and weight loss. So I used my own photos, statistics, facts, and stories to do so. As mentioned before I have now met others who also have lost weight by eating all-organic foods too. But this sequel will be written so that YOUR stories, facts, statistics, and photos will convince even more people how this new lifestyle is so easy and works!

You can also email TheEasiestDiet@aol.com any questions, comments, complaints, criticisms, or complements concerning this book and the program.

Also if you have any additional orders for this book you can email them to the same address and place your orders there too. Reduced prices will be available for those who have already purchased the book and want additional copies, or for those who order five or more copies at the same time.

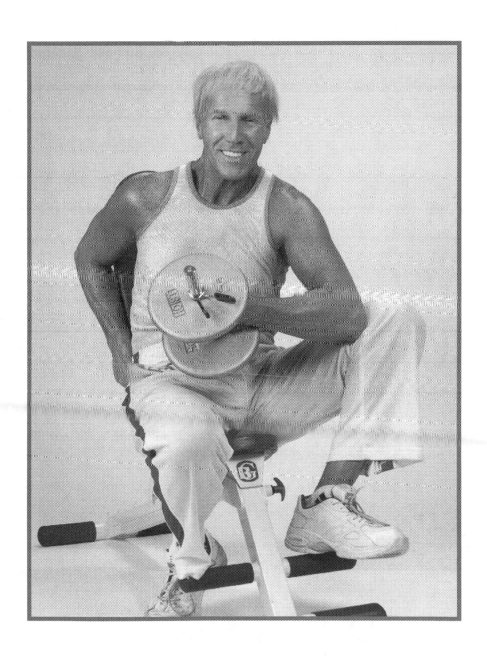

# CHAPTER 18

# Part III- The Special Charts/Logs Section

Another special feature of this book for you is this next section which I call the Pocket "Yellow Jacket".....the buzz you hear is not that of a wasp. The buzz you hear are the important points section of this "Yellow Jacket".

It contains logs and charts which can help your motivation and also help you reach your goals. Also whenever you hit a snag, it can help you discover why.

I have compiled here some charts and logs that you can use to record your efforts. I have included these sets twice in the same order: logs 1-5 followed by the Terrific Tips Toward Total Health section. I have done this so that you can print out additional copies and use these and keep a file on your progress. You could even tear out the second set of these from the book and leave the first set right in the book as the last pages of the book. Use all of them, or just whichever ones you find useful.

1) <u>Progress Chart for Your New Lifestyle</u>
This first chart you should DEFINITELY want to use! It is your total progress chart with the key measurements of success you will have achieved! You will want to frame this chart! You start with the date you initiate the new lifestyle and put your original starting measurements on it: height, weight, waist size, cholesterol readings, and triglyceride readings. I only have the height listed there (as obviously your height will not change due

to this lifestyle) just so that you can research different charts that are published to see possible "ideal" weights for certain heights and certain body types.

Then there is the section where you list these same statistics after 4 months on the program, 5 months on the program, and finally 6 months on the program. Most people will achieve their ideal goals somewhere between 4-6 months. Congratulations!! You will see the results. Now frame this sheet!!! And you WILL stay on this lifestyle program because it is indeed: The Easiest Diet in the World...and It Works!

2) Daily Total Program Chart

On this chart you can put your total food intake of all your meals and snacks, your cardio walking regimen, and your weight training workout if it falls on that day. All of them can be written by you on the same daily total program sheet. You could then keep these files and have your whole year's progress charted. Then YOU could even write a better book than I did because you will know exactly where and when you lost your poundage!

3) Weekly Meals Log

On this chart you log every meal you have for a whole week's time. The main purpose of this would be that if you noticed you had gained 2 or more pounds during the last week, you could then look back at the weekly meals log and discover why you had done so. I do not specifically keep such a written log myself right now, but if I notice myself gaining closer toward the upper limit of my ideal weight, I think back to what I had the last week and usually realize what food item(s) I was eating too much of that week. It would be a lot easier for me to do this if I kept this weekly food log myself to correct any bad habits I sometimes fall into...like my ice cream cravings!

4) <u>Weekly Walking Log</u>

On it you chart out your daily cardio walks for a whole week and make notes on any changes your routes should entail for the future. You will want to see how many different routes you can walk during a year's time also! I even give a place for those of you who are concerned about the mileage you walk so you can put your distance traveled with each daily walk.

5) <u>Weekly Workout Log</u>

This is what you can use to keep track of your weight training workouts if you choose to add this third component of the New Lifestyle Change talked about in this book. There are places for each exercise name, the number of pounds you are using on that exercise, the number of sets you do, and the number of repetitions done during each set.

6)

# Terrific
# Tips
# Toward
# Total Health

Yes, here in quick short form are all of the most important concepts to keep in mind about this New Lifestyle Change. Keep this handy and follow these guidelines as much as possible! I have included this section twice, each time at the end of this logs/charts section. This is so that you can remove the last copy of it and place it on your refrigerator with a magnet to refer to each of these key points of the book.

# PROGRESS CHART FOR YOUR NEW LIFESTYLE

START DATE: _____

<u>INITIAL STATISTICS</u>:

Height: _____

Weight: _____

Waist Size: _____

Cholesterol:   LDL (bad): _____

                 HDL (good): _____

Triglycerides: _____

<u>PROGRESS REPORT</u>

<u>AFTER</u>: 4 MThs: Date: _____ 5 MThs: Date: _____ 6 MThs: Date:_____

Height: _____      _____      _____

Weight: _____      _____      _____

Waist Size: _____      _____      _____

Cholesterol:
  LDL (bad): _____      _____      _____

    HDL (good): _____      _____      _____

Triglycerides: _____      _____      _____

# DAILY TOTAL PROGRAM CHART

DATE: _____ DAY OF WEEK: _____

<u>MEALS</u>

BREAKFAST: One full grapefruit with organic sweetener PLUS:

_____

MID MORNING SNACK: _____

_____

LUNCH: _____

_____

MID-AFTERNOON SNACK: _____

_____

SUPPER: _____

_____

<u>CARDIO WALK</u>: TIME BEGUN: _____ TIME ENDED: _____

PLACE: _____

COMMENTS: _____

_____

<u>WEIGHT TRAINING</u>:

EXERCISE: _____ # LBS. USED: _____

# SETS DONE: _____ # REPS PER SET: _____

EXERCISE: _____ # LBS. USED: _____

# SETS DONE: _____ # REPS PER SET: _____

EXERCISE: _____ # LBS. USED: _____

# SETS DONE: _____ # REPS PER SET: _____

# WEEKLY MEALS LOG

WEEK OF: _____ WEIGHT: _____

SUNDAY: BREAKFAST: _____

_____

MID-AM SNACK: _____

LUNCH: _____

_____

MID-PM SNACK: _____

DINNER: _____

_____

MONDAY: BREAKFAST: _____

_____

MID-AM SNACK: _____

LUNCH: _____

_____

MID-PM SNACK: _____

DINNER: _____

_____


TUESDAY: BREAKFAST: _____

_____

MID-AM SNACK: _____

LUNCH: _____

_____

MID-PM SNACK: _____

DINNER: _____

_____

WEDNESDAY: BREAKFAST: _____

_____

MID-AM SNACK: _____

LUNCH: _____

_____

MID-PM SNACK: _____

DINNER: _____

_____


THURSDAY: BREAKFAST:_____

_____

MID-AM SNACK: _____

LUNCH: _____

_____

MID-PM SNACK: _____

DINNER: _____

_____

FRIDAY: BREAKFAST:_____

_____

MID-AM SNACK: _____

LUNCH: _____

_____

MID-PM SNACK: _____

DINNER: _____

_____


SATURDAY: BREAKFAST:_____

_____

MID-AM SNACK: _____

LUNCH: _____

_____

MID-PM SNACK: _____

DINNER: _____

_____

# WEEKLY WALKING LOG

WEEK OF _____

SUNDAY: PLACE _____

TIME STARTED: _____ TIME ENDED: _____ DISTANCE:_____

COMMENTS: _____

_____

_____

MONDAY: PLACE _____

TIME STARTED: _____ TIME ENDED: _____ DISTANCE:_____

COMMENTS: _____

_____

_____

TUESDAY: PLACE _____

TIME STARTED: _____ TIME ENDED: _____ DISTANCE:_____

COMMENTS: _____

_____

_____

WEDNESDAY: PLACE _____

TIME STARTED: _____ TIME ENDED: _____ DISTANCE:_____

COMMENTS: _____

_____

_____


THURSDAY: PLACE _____

TIME STARTED: _____ TIME ENDED: _____ DISTANCE:_____

COMMENTS: _____

_____

_____


FRIDAY: PLACE _____

TIME STARTED: _____ TIME ENDED: _____ DISTANCE:_____

COMMENTS: _____

_____

_____


SATURDAY: PLACE _____

TIME STARTED: _____ TIME ENDED: _____ DISTANCE:_____

COMMENTS: _____

_____

_____

# WEEKLY WORKOUT LOG

DATE: _____

EXERCISE: _____ # LBS. USED: _____

    # SETS: _____ # REPS: _____

COMMENTS: _____

_____

_____

EXERCISE: _____ # LBS. USED: _____

    # SETS: _____ # REPS: _____

COMMENTS: _____

_____

_____

EXERCISE: _____ # LBS. USED: _____

    # SETS: _____ # REPS: _____

COMMENTS: _____

_____

_____

DATE: _____

EXERCISE: _____ # LBS. USED: _____

    # SETS: _____ # REPS: _____

COMMENTS: _____

_____

_____


EXERCISE: _____ # LBS. USED: _____

    # SETS: _____ # REPS: _____

COMMENTS: _____

_____

_____


EXERCISE: _____ # LBS. USED: _____

    # SETS: _____ # REPS: _____

COMMENTS: _____

_____

_____

DATE: _____

EXERCISE: _____ # LBS. USED: _____

     # SETS: _____ # REPS: _____

COMMENTS: _____

_____

_____

EXERCISE: _____ # LBS. USED: _____

     # SETS: _____ # REPS: _____

COMMENTS: _____

_____

_____

EXERCISE: _____ # LBS. USED: _____

     # SETS: _____ # REPS: _____

COMMENTS: _____

_____

_____

DATE: _____

EXERCISE: _____ # LBS. USED: _____

    # SETS: _____ # REPS: _____

COMMENTS: _____

_____

_____

EXERCISE: _____ # LBS. USED: _____

    # SETS: _____ # REPS: _____

COMMENTS: _____

_____

_____

EXERCISE: _____ # LBS. USED: _____

    # SETS: _____ # REPS: _____

COMMENTS: _____

_____

_____

# Terrific Tips Toward Total Health

Do NOT weigh yourself until at least ONE month has passed {2 months if you can wait that long even}!

Then weigh yourself every week: same time, place, scale, amount of clothes on.

Eat nothing but ORGANIC foods/drink all the time using ALL ORGANIC ingredients: condiments, dressings, etc.

If you need to save money, you can buy non-organic raw produce: fruits and vegetables.

Be sure though that all processed food you buy/eat (packaged, frozen, cans) are ORGANIC!

All dairy, meats, and eggs, should be organic with no hormones or preservatives used and with only free-range, grass-fed animals.

TRY NOT to have anything to eat 2-3 hours before you go to bed each night also.

As more people buy/use organic products, the prices will drop.

To save money, try regular super markets, Costco and then health food stores in that order for purchasing organic foods.

You should lose 10-20% of your body weight within 4-6 months of starting this program.

You do not need to be concerned with the amount of calories necessarily, but keep track of your food intake by using the weekly meal log provided.

You do not need to be concerned with the amount of fat or carbohydrates you are eating either.

You will reach your "ideal" weight after one year in the program. If you notice that you have gained more than 3 pounds from your "ideal" weight in any particular week, look carefully at what you ate the last week and make the appropriate changes in overeating of that item.

Remember organic foods do not have the additives and preservatives that make you "addictive" to eating more than you want/need/should eat.

Your cholesterol, blood pressure and triglyceride levels should all improve and be in "normal" healthy range within one year of your program start.

You will have higher self-esteem and definitely be motivated to stay on this program the rest of your life!

When on vacations get a room with a microwave and small refrigerator and buy/eat organic foods. Go to organic restaurants.

Try WholeFoodFarmacy's Tri-Decathlon Delux Diet Loss Program to cleanse out your body once a year.

Read labels on "natural" foods to be sure they contain no preservatives or additives and no chemicals to be "essentially organic". Then you could purchase them if they pass that "test".

Do one hour of continuous cardio training every day: walking, swimming, or bicycling.

Use ideas in this book to vary the paths by incorporating your cardio walk into your daily schedule of what you are doing/where you are going.

Do "hap-hazard" walks in cities or strange areas by going North and East, OR North and West, OR South and East, OR South and West and then coming back to your starting point in opposite directions the last half hour.

On your daily walks bring the following: a water bottle, a reward (suggested=an organic apple), a handkerchief or tissues, your ID, and a cell phone.

The use of the Precor Elliptic Cross Trainer or Mountain Climber Machines is fine, but not tread mill!

Just be sure you do continuous movement in your cardio for one hour every day!

The least important, but still good component of the program is to do weight training with machines on your upper body and abs. Use low weight and many reps and gradually add on the weight week by week or month by month.

For helpful supplements use D4 Thermal Shock capsules and AMP Amplified N.O. Loaded from GNC.

# PROGRESS CHART FOR YOUR NEW LIFESTYLE

START DATE: _____

INITIAL STATISTICS:

Height: _____

Weight: _____

Waist Size: _____

Cholesterol:   LDL (bad): _____

                 HDL (good): _____

Triglycerides: _____

PROGRESS REPORT

AFTER: 4 MThs: Date: _____ 5 MThs: Date: _____ 6 MThs: Date:_____

Height: _____      _____      _____

Weight: _____      _____      _____

Waist Size: _____      _____      _____

Cholesterol:
  LDL (bad): _____      _____      _____

  HDL (good): _____      _____      _____

Triglycerides: _____      _____      _____

# DAILY TOTAL PROGRAM CHART

DATE: _____ DAY OF WEEK: _____

<u>MEALS</u>

BREAKFAST: One full grapefruit with organic sweetener PLUS:

_____

MID MORNING SNACK: _____

_____

LUNCH: _____

_____

MID-AFTERNOON SNACK: _____

_____

SUPPER: _____

_____

<u>CARDIO WALK</u>: TIME BEGUN: _____ TIME ENDED: _____

PLACE: _____

COMMENTS: _____

_____

<u>WEIGHT TRAINING</u>:

EXERCISE: _____ # LBS. USED: _____

# SETS DONE: _____ # REPS PER SET: _____

EXERCISE: _____ # LBS. USED: _____

# SETS DONE: _____ # REPS PER SET: _____

EXERCISE: _____ # LBS. USED: _____

# SETS DONE: _____ # REPS PER SET: _____

# WEEKLY MEALS LOG

WEEK OF: _____ WEIGHT: _____

SUNDAY: BREAKFAST: _____

_____

MID-AM SNACK: _____

LUNCH: _____

_____

MID-PM SNACK: _____

DINNER: _____

_____

MONDAY: BREAKFAST: _____

_____

MID-AM SNACK: _____

LUNCH: _____

_____

MID-PM SNACK: _____

DINNER: _____

_____


TUESDAY: BREAKFAST: _____

_____

MID-AM SNACK: _____

LUNCH: _____

_____

MID-PM SNACK: _____

DINNER: _____

_____

WEDNESDAY: BREAKFAST: _____

_____

MID-AM SNACK: _____

LUNCH: _____

_____

MID-PM SNACK: _____

DINNER: _____

_____


THURSDAY: BREAKFAST:_____

_____

MID-AM SNACK: _____

LUNCH: _____

_____

MID-PM SNACK: _____

DINNER: _____

_____

FRIDAY: BREAKFAST:_____

_____

MID-AM SNACK: _____

LUNCH: _____

_____

MID-PM SNACK: _____

DINNER: _____

_____


SATURDAY: BREAKFAST:_____

_____

MID-AM SNACK: _____

LUNCH: _____

_____

MID-PM SNACK: _____

DINNER: _____

_____

# WEEKLY WALKING LOG

WEEK OF _____

<u>SUNDAY:</u> PLACE _____

TIME STARTED: _____ TIME ENDED: _____ DISTANCE:_____

COMMENTS: _____

_____

_____

<u>MONDAY:</u> PLACE _____

TIME STARTED: _____ TIME ENDED: _____ DISTANCE:_____

COMMENTS: _____

_____

_____

<u>TUESDAY:</u> PLACE _____

TIME STARTED: _____ TIME ENDED: _____ DISTANCE:_____

COMMENTS: _____

_____

_____

WEDNESDAY: PLACE _____

TIME STARTED: _____ TIME ENDED: _____ DISTANCE:_____

COMMENTS: _____

_____

_____

THURSDAY: PLACE _____

TIME STARTED: _____ TIME ENDED: _____ DISTANCE:_____

COMMENTS: _____

_____

_____

FRIDAY: PLACE _____

TIME STARTED: _____ TIME ENDED: _____ DISTANCE:_____

COMMENTS: _____

_____

_____

SATURDAY: PLACE _____

TIME STARTED: _____ TIME ENDED: _____ DISTANCE:_____

COMMENTS: _____

_____

_____

# WEEKLY WORKOUT LOG

DATE: _____

EXERCISE: _____ # LBS. USED: _____

    # SETS: _____ # REPS: _____

COMMENTS: _____

_____

_____

EXERCISE: _____ # LBS. USED: _____

    # SETS: _____ # REPS: _____

COMMENTS: _____

_____

_____

EXERCISE: _____ # LBS. USED: _____

    # SETS: _____ # REPS: _____

COMMENTS: _____

_____

_____

DATE: _____

EXERCISE: _____ # LBS. USED: _____

    # SETS: _____ # REPS: _____

COMMENTS: _____

_____

_____

EXERCISE: _____ # LBS. USED: _____

    # SETS: _____ # REPS: _____

COMMENTS: _____

_____

_____

EXERCISE: _____ # LBS. USED: _____

    # SETS: _____ # REPS: _____

COMMENTS: _____

_____

_____

DATE: _____

EXERCISE: _____ # LBS. USED: _____

    # SETS: _____ # REPS: _____

COMMENTS: _____

_____

_____

EXERCISE: _____ # LBS. USED: _____

    # SETS: _____ # REPS: _____

COMMENTS: _____

_____

_____

EXERCISE: _____ # LBS. USED: _____

    # SETS: _____ # REPS: _____

COMMENTS: _____

_____

_____

DATE: _____

EXERCISE: _____ # LBS. USED: _____

    # SETS: _____ # REPS: _____

COMMENTS: _____

_____

_____

EXERCISE: _____ # LBS. USED: _____

    # SETS: _____ # REPS: _____

COMMENTS: _____

_____

_____

EXERCISE: _____ # LBS. USED: _____

    # SETS: _____ # REPS: _____

COMMENTS: _____

_____

_____

# Terrific Tips Toward Total Health

Do NOT weigh yourself until at least ONE month has passed {2 months if you can wait that long even}!

Then weigh yourself every week: same time, place, scale, amount of clothes on.

Eat nothing but ORGANIC foods/drink all the time using ALL ORGANIC ingredients: condiments, dressings, etc.

If you need to save money, you can buy non-organic raw produce: fruits and vegetables.

Be sure though that all processed food you buy/eat (packaged, frozen, cans) are ORGANIC!

All dairy, meats, and eggs, should be organic with no hormones or preservatives used and with only free-range, grass-fed animals.

TRY NOT to have anything to eat 2-3 hours before you go to bed each night also.

As more people buy/use organic products, the prices will drop.

To save money, try regular super markets, Costco and then health food stores in that order for purchasing organic foods.

You should lose 10-20% of your body weight within 4-6 months of starting this program.

You do not need to be concerned with the amount of calories necessarily, but keep track of your food intake by using the weekly meal log provided.

You do not need to be concerned with the amount of fat or carbohydrates you are eating either.

You will reach your "ideal" weight after one year in the program. If you notice that you have gained more than 3 pounds from your "ideal" weight in any particular week, look carefully at what you ate the last week and make the appropriate changes in overeating of that item.

Remember organic foods do not have the additives and preservatives that make you "addictive" to eating more than you want/need/should eat.

Your cholesterol, blood pressure and triglyceride levels should all improve and be in "normal" healthy range within one year of your program start.

You will have higher self-esteem and definitely be motivated to stay on this program the rest of your life!

When on vacations get a room with a microwave and small refrigerator and buy/eat organic foods. Go to organic restaurants.

Try WholeFoodFarmacy's Tri-Decathlon Delux Diet Loss Program to cleanse out your body once a year.

Read labels on "natural" foods to be sure they contain no preservatives or additives and no chemicals to be "essentially organic". Then you could purchase them if they pass that "test".

Do one hour of continuous cardio training every day: walking, swimming, or bicycling.

Use ideas in this book to vary the paths by incorporating your cardio walk into your daily schedule of what you are doing/where you are going.

Do "hap-hazard" walks in cities or strange areas by going North and East, OR North and West, OR South and East, OR South and West and then coming back to your starting point in opposite directions the last half hour.

On your daily walks bring the following: a water bottle, a reward (suggested=an organic apple), a handkerchief or tissues, your ID, and a cell phone.

The use of the Precor Elliptic Cross Trainer or Mountain Climber Machines is fine, but not tread mill!

Just be sure you do continuous movement in your cardio for one hour every day!

The least important, but still good component of the program is to do weight training with machines on your upper body and abs. Use low weight and many reps and gradually add on the weight week by week or month by month.

For helpful supplements use D4 Thermal Shock capsules and AMP Amplified N.O. Loaded from GNC.

To get that final inch removed or for that "finishing touch" you can check into the use of Lipo-Dissolve Technique.